CANCER

Reflections on life with cancer...
and finding the good in any challenge.

Author Debi Hampton

WestBow Press books may be ordered through
booksellers or by contacting:

WestBow Press
A Division of Thomas Nelson & Zondervan
1663 Liberty Drive
Bloomington, IN 47403
www.westbowpress.com
1 (866) 928-1240

Because of the dynamic nature of the Internet, any web addresses or
links contained in this book may have changed since publication and
may no longer be valid. The views expressed in this work are solely those
of the author and do not necessarily reflect the views of the publisher,
and the publisher hereby disclaims any responsibility for them.

Cover image: Photo: Nicole Hampton, Enhance: Debi Hampton

Scripture taken from the Holy Bible, NEW INTERNATIONAL
VERSION®. Copyright © 1973, 1978, 1984, 2011 by Biblica,
Inc. All rights reserved worldwide. Used by permission. NEW
INTERNATIONAL VERSION® and NIV® are registered trademarks
of Biblica, Inc. Use of either trademark for the offering of goods or
services requires the prior written consent of Biblica US, Inc.

This book is a work of non-fiction. Unless otherwise noted, the author
and the publisher make no explicit guarantees as to the accuracy of
the information contained in this book and in some cases, names
of people and places have been altered to protect their privacy.

ISBN: 978-1-5127-3139-2 (sc)
ISBN: 978-1-5127-3140-8 (hc)
ISBN: 978-1-5127-3138-5 (e)

Library of Congress Control Number: 2016902946

Print information available on the last page.

WestBow Press rev. date: 3/9/2016

... to the future ...

Through life experiences, and seeing God in them despite myself, I have come to not only look back for God in my life, but to look forward for Him on my continued journey.

My expectations have shifted. God is not only a belief in my head, but a presence in my heart. He is not visible by sight in front of me, but His Spirit abounds within me.

Now... I am looking upward and onward to the future, knowing that God is with me... no longer wondering... fully convicted in my heart that He has always been there. I am excited for a new day and what He will offer. :)

almightystory@gmail.com

Has God empowered you to be mighty through a life challenge? I look forward to reading about your journey of faith and fulfillment through belief in God, His Word and His presence in your life. If you are led to do so, please email me your story.

www.wrapinlove.com

This website is brand new, as is this venture of God empowering me to connect with you via this book. Check it out. It will be a work in progress, updated as I am led to do so. Please contact me through the website if you have questions about the website or suggestions as to how to make it better. We are in this together!

SOURCES

biblegateway.com
New International Version (NIV)

dictionary.com

prb.org

··· *dedicated to Him* ···

*This is the simplest passage to write. I am humbled,
encouraged and so grateful for God's presence!
My life is influenced by many wise and amazing people,
and my journey would not be as such without them!*

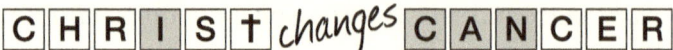

This is a good life! I am free from the burdens of others and those I put upon myself. This book is a prime example of this, as God is my lead. No way would I have set out to write a book. God, instead, gave me words to write in haste on found scraps of paper. This became a passion. God spoke to my heart, but none of it would have been possible had my life gone differently in any way. The cancer gave me a forum. Freelancing gave me the opportunity, both with time and knowledge. My family and friends shared in the writing of my experiences, as they were instrumental in the creation of them.

Many thanks go to my mom, Leona Prushing, who has faced many challenges, while placing her life in His hands. Aaron's parents, Tom and Nina Lee Hampton, have also strongly impacted my life with His presence. This book is dedicated to the lives that created mine, especially to our parents who have been there for us through thick and thin. There have been so many times when breaking down emotionally was inevitable, but they were there to pick us up, to care for us, to pray with us, to encourage us through one more difficult day. God provides. He always has, and He always will, if we put our trust in Him. I am so thankful for God's gift of amazing parents!

I pray that our kids will continue to know the love and greatness of God's promises through the influence of our parents, our church family, and other family and friends! What a glorious day when I *truly* realized how much God loves Nicole, Nathan and Noelle. We love them beyond words, and God cares so much more! God has this much love for every human being! May we all keep God in our hearts, with His spirit emulating from our souls. We welcome His return, and ask Him to guide our feet as we walk, our hands as we work, our ears as we listen for Him, our eyes as we look for Him in action, our minds as we think upon and pray with Him through the good and the difficult, and our hearts as we live our faith in Him until that day.

Reflections Include

⋯ *the cancer word* ⋯

Hearing the diagnosis of cancer is beyond difficult.
We have already wondered and worried the inevitable
what-if scenarios as we await our test results.
Then it is confirmed.

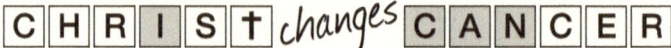

`C` `H` `R` `I` `S` `†` *changes* `C` `A` `N` `C` `E` `R`

The memory is still vivid in my mind. The deep sadness overcame me in my car after dropping our daughter at a soccer clinic in Dublin. My endocrinologist had called to tell me the biopsy from my left thyroid nodule aspiration had come back questionable with cancer. He recommended surgery to remove the left half of my thyroid, followed by radioactive iodine treatment to eradicate any remaining thyroid cells that could be cancerous.

I held it together until she left the car. Then tears flowed and my heart ached for the certain physical and emotional pain that would soon enter our world. It seemed so daunting. Due to my limited knowledge of cancer, the "c" word seemed like a death sentence. I am now a seven-year survivor with a positive prognosis, including ongoing checks for life. Cancer is no longer about death for me. We will all die at sometime by something. It is about the life we live in the time we have, no matter how long that is.

The words he said via phone on that sunny evening on June 11, 2008 would **confirm** that my life was about to change forever.

Even though the grief of the cancer news briefly overshadowed my certain belief in God, I soon was back in prayer with the knowledge that His light would lead me through a very draining and frightful time in our lives. We would face my fears together, and He would bring comfort to my soul. No joke... it was hard. Tears come even now at the memory of the dark and sad hours. But there was joy too.

Psalm 23:4
Even though I walk through the darkest valley, I will fear no evil, for you are with me; your rod and your staff, they comfort me.

What is the story of your diagnosis or traumatic news?

_____

_____

_____

_____

_____

_____

_____

_____

_____

_____

_____

_____

_____

_____

_____

_____

_____

_____

... so many unknowns ...

Even though my faith in God was sure,
cancer would still challenge me in many ways.
There were questions to ask God, to ask my doctors,
to ask my family and to ask myself.

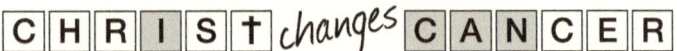

Why me? How did this happen? Will I die? What will Aaron, my husband, and our children do without me? They were young. Noelle was a fragile two years old. Nathan took it all to heart at six, and Nicole was a brave big sister at ten. How will we pay for the surgery and the treatment? Will I be sick or lose my hair? The fear of the unknown smacked me square in the face. We needed **clarity**.

After the initial shock, discussions with doctors, hours of research online, and daily, deep, heart-felt prayer, we came to grips with my cancer, my treatment and the winding path that was before us.

As with all bad news and difficulties, it is harder in the beginning. Like a nasty, bleeding wound, that needs healing. Our minds and bodies were raw with pain. But it was okay. This too would pass. Aaron and I used to joke that certain unpleasant phases in the kids lives would eventually end, like sleepless nights, illnesses and poopy diapers. We made it through each phase together, better after all.

Cancer is quite a bit different, I agree. But there are analogies that can be drawn. Each step in your cancer journey is a phase that will pass. Things will **change**, they always do. Some better. Some worse.

Our job is to embrace whatever comes our way, hand in hand with God, and held up by our support systems. Make every day a new day to make a difference to someone. Share the love of God somehow, somewhere. Keep our heads high, stand tall, and keep a smile of peace on our face, knowing God is always with us.

Deuteronomy 31:6

Be strong and courageous. Do not be afraid or terrified because of them, for the Lord your God goes with you; He will never leave you nor forsake you.

What questions did you ask yourself and others?

_____

_____

_____

_____

_____

_____

_____

_____

_____

_____

_____

_____

_____

_____

_____

_____

_____

_____

... a special calling ...

*This journey of surviving cancer continues to
change my life and to strengthen my faith every day.
God knows our hearts, our joys, our concerns, our fears
and our pain... like a parent knows their own child's.*

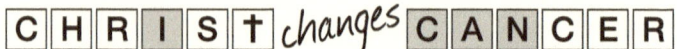

I recently learned of Jeremy Camp's loss of his first wife to cancer. He sings, "He Knows," to share his pain and his story of praise to a God who wants to know us intimately. "He is near to the broken hearted, every tear, He knows..." As our spiritual parent, He is right there beside us through the good and the bad, but we have to open our hearts to His existence and His amazing promise.

A year into my treatment, my endo asked me if I was "managing" my cancer. I thought it odd, especially because he knew my high anxiety. The next year, he asked the same. Even though it has not been an easy journey, the truth is, I *have* embraced my cancer as a special **calling** to be strong and to continue here on earth doing whatever, wherever and for however long God leads me. He knows the number of hairs on my head. How cool is that?

So until we meet again, we cherish the memories of all of those who have passed before us. People die every day, and we must find the strength to carry on in their absence. Death is not the end.

Dictionary.com says a "survivor" is one who functions or prospers in spite of opposition, hardship or setbacks. Surviving is the ability to push through and find a way to keep going. Cancer is not a choice, but we choose how we fight. Cancer is a calling to trust God and to share your story. Celebrate overcoming challenges and find joy in His blessings. Look for God in your life. Once you start seeing Him, you will know He has always been here and will always be.

John 1:1-3

In the beginning was the Word, and the Word was with God, and the Word was God. He was with God in the beginning. Through Him all things were made, without Him nothing was made...

What is different in your life since diagnosis?

_____

_____

_____

_____

_____

_____

_____

_____

_____

_____

_____

_____

_____

_____

_____

_____

... joined the club ...

*As a survivor, we are a member of the "cancer club."
Honorary members are friends and family that endure
the life-threatening illness with us and step into our lives
to keep us going. You are not alone in any challenge.*

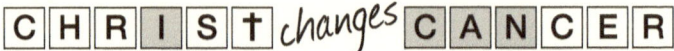

I thank God daily for our family and friends. They made meals, sent cards and emails, called to check on us and prayed with us through it all. What a blessing! **Cuddle** on the couch and hug often, even when feeling lousy. I heard a story of a man who wore a "FREE HUGS" sign on the street corner. A homeless woman watched others accept his free gift and asked what the sign said, as she could not read. A simple hug was given to lift the spirits of a woman not hugged in many years. It brought comfort, encouragement and hope to both.

Part of healing is coming to terms with the cancer, making a plan and staying positive. Find the good in people and in your circumstances every minute of every day. Rejoice in joining the club, in not being alone in the fight. There were days I simply felt horrid. Other days were emotionally draining and physically exhausting for myself and my family. Thank you God for the simple things, like smiles and hugs, hands to hold and quiet moments when nothing hurts. In your darkest hours, purposefully place yourself in a place of peace and calm. Sit with God, joyful in still being alive and for all He has given.

Ponder the day when you will tell your story for the first time to a cancer newbie, **cheerful** and encouraging as you guide them to God for the journey ahead. Make a conscious choice right now to keep your glass half full, not half empty. I stumble every day, but God is with me as I get up and try again. Thank Him for the difficult and the easy, both integral parts of who we are. I am thankful for my cancer.

I Thessalonians 5:16-18

Rejoice always, pray continually, give thanks in all circumstances; for this is God's will for you in Christ Jesus.

What makes you feel thankful and blessed?

_____

_____

_____

_____

_____

_____

_____

_____

_____

_____

_____

_____

_____

_____

_____

_____

_____

... a purposeful story ...

Being a survivor of any illness or traumatic event is a reason to share the story. Once you have lived it, you know the fear, the sadness, the questions and the challenges that lie ahead. Reach out to others and share.

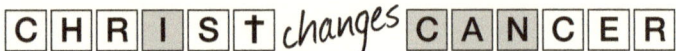

C H R I S † *changes* C A N C E R

Christ died for all of us to take away our sin. His grace covers our weakness. God wants us to live for Him, as He died for us. Pray for ways to praise God and to share His gospel of love, as you share your own journey of illness, treatment and recovery. Talk about **courage**.

Survivors are like sick plants, broken and wilted. With nutrients, water, sun and lots of love, we look forward to blossoming into beautiful flowers once again, if even for only a short time.

Our kids are all so different and yet incredibly wonderful each in their own way. It is so rewarding and joyful to hear their stories of success, fun and joy. Noelle's excitement of a new dance in ballet, Nathan's wonder about the glowing minerals in science class and Nicole's enthusiastic reflection on a good game of soccer.

What amazing gifts from God! The happy stories are fun and fantastic! Share your joys, as small as they may be, throughout your cancer experience. I felt joy after surgery, knowing that the first step of treatment was complete. The surgery was a success with all of my thyroid removed. The nausea from the pain and anesthesia meds made me sick, but did not kill me. Bumpy road, but we made it to our first destination!

Find your wings in the strong moments. Fly high, and then soar with God when you are down and just need to make it through the day. "Suck it up buttercup," I would say to myself. Take comfort in the Bible, with writings of triumphant journeys and messages of hope.

Isaiah 40:31

But those who hope in the Lord will renew their strength. They will soar on wings like eagles; they will run and not grow weary, they will walk and not be faint.

What can you do in the life of another?

_____

_____

_____

_____

_____

_____

_____

_____

_____

_____

_____

_____

_____

_____

_____

_____

_____

_____

… no easy button …

*Looking back, there are several times in my life that
God was working even though I was unaware.
He knows our hearts, our desires, our hopes and our
dreams. Our Father loves us more than we can imagine.*

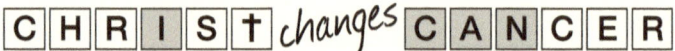

We may not understand our struggle, but there is meaning, hope and love. The act of surviving hardship is rewarding and changes the heart in positive ways. Without the hard, there would be no reward. No pain, no gain. God walks with us through the valley of darkness.

Pray for a heart of **calm** surrender to His will. God never leaves us, even if our faith is shaken. Whether you unquestionably believe in God's existence because of life experience, or you simply have hope in a higher being, look for Him in your life and the lives of those around you. I look back on my life, and see God all over it, even though I was oblivious at the time. He has blessed us abundantly!

The pain, guilt, shame and doubt of being date raped my senior year in college is just a memory now. A difficult time when my friend then, husband now, would care for and defend me through the confusion of the drug given and the emotional toll caused by another man. The turmoil of that time has been quieted, replaced by peace. Even though Aaron and I have had our share of life struggles, I believe God has always been with us, and I thank Him for my best friend.

A baby born to our drug addict friend was saved by God. Now four years old, God's plan for this sweet boy began over 15 years ago when Aaron and I met his birth mom through Big Brothers Big Sisters. She sadly continued to self-destruct and put her child's life in danger. We fostered him until his adoption to his forever family, surrounded by God's love. A difficult journey, but God knew His plan.

Romans 8:28

And we know that in all things God works for the good of those who love him, who have been called according to his purpose.

What hardships have changed you for the better?

_____

_____

_____

_____

_____

_____

_____

_____

_____

_____

_____

_____

_____

_____

_____

_____

... redefine our failure ...

The stress of cancer is immense, physically and emotionally. After especially difficult times, dealing with treatment and finances, I remember feeling guilty for our apparent failures. There were days I nearly lost my mind.

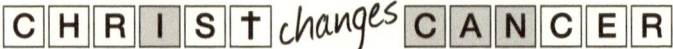

The pain of sadness, frustration and failure exploding from within, to envelope those closest to me, even as they dealt with their own pain. Even today, fear and doubt will rise up with finances, time constraints, life stresses and ongoing cancer concerns. We make positive progress every day, but it is easy to fall into the "want it now" trap. I know my family still loves me, even when I mess up and vent unfairly. It is hard to keep a balance. God helps. He reminds us to be **content**, to seek His strength, to trust Him and to be patient.

Medical bills since 2008 even with insurance, plus what we already owed from other life circumstances, was a toxic combo. Every year, though, we are closer to being debt-free. Keep trying every day, even if you feel like you are failing. Financial freedom would likely not happen for us if it were not *for the cancer*. It forced us to face our debt reality. Aaron has a great job and insurance, and we welcome a positive financial future. We are also blessed to have parents who graciously assist us with bills. God provides all that we *need*.

We have failed in many ways, but the failure truly sets us free. Dictionary.com defines "failure" as an act or instance proving unsuccessful. Let us redefine the word failure, as an act or instance of giving us the ability to redirect, change or embrace whatever we strive to succeed within. Learn from mistakes and push forth! Freely apologize to those you hurt. Everyone on this planet has sinned, but One. We are not alone. Stand up again, and **carry** on.

Philippians 4:12-13

I have learned the secret of being content in any and every situation, whether well fed or hungry, whether living in plenty or in want. I can do all things through Him who gives me strength.

What have you endured that ended well?

_____

_____

_____

_____

_____

_____

_____

_____

_____

_____

_____

_____

_____

_____

_____

_____

··· *find your happy* ···

Make determined and positive goals for the future.
Look at short-term and long-term goals that will set
you up for success regarding your cancer, overall health,
family and friends, career, and living a good life!

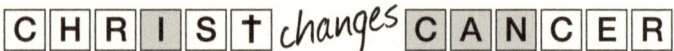

Why waller in the negativity of despair and fear? Stand up tall, wipe off the negative "goo," take hold of God's hand and figure out how you are going to make it through this defining moment. I have tripped and fallen back into the mud several times. I have splattered mud on my family and friends. They kept praying with me and looking up with me to see the sun peeking through the clouds. Do not wait for happiness to find you. God is always there, just as is the sun, even if our vision is blocked by the rain and clouds in the storm. Joy is a choice. I love the movie "Unconditional." The main character is faced with the death of her husband, but she learns to live again.

Never give up hope. HOPE means "Hold On Pain Ends." Fight for what you want, while asking God for guidance in deciding what that should be. Keep positive thoughts in your brain and happy words on the tip of your tongue, while you fight for a ***cure***. Make a difference to someone this very day! Share a joke, simply smile or compliment your nurse, as they serve you in treatment and recovery. God is big. He wants us to dream big. My new favorite quote is, "If your dreams don't scare you, they're not big enough."

Church families are wonderful places to find support and to give back. After all, this family is an extension of God's spirit. I view our church as a hospital, a place for spiritual healing and rejuvenation. Seek out a ***church*** home or a group of believers. We have felt much love and encouragement from our church family.

Hebrews 10:24-25

And let us consider how we may spur one another on toward love and good deeds, not giving up meeting together, as some are in the habit of doing, but encouraging one another.

What short-term and long-term goals have you set?

_____

_____

_____

_____

_____

_____

_____

_____

_____

_____

_____

_____

_____

_____

_____

⋯ *give it all* ⋯

*God provides! It may not be when or where or how
we think He should provide, but He does. Looking back,
I think now, "How did I not see what He was doing?
Why did I doubt Him? Now I understand why."*

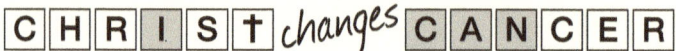

Take a lemon, add some sugar and make some lemonade. Face the issue, the problem, the illness; add prayer, positive thoughts, encouraging words; and run straight into the fear, doubt, worry and pain. At least you will know what you are facing. Who knows, maybe it will not be as bad as you initially thought. Find a way to **cope**.

God wants us to give it all to Him and to let Him take care of it. Of course, He wants us to participate and to do our own part. But ultimately the solution will come from Him. Even when it is tough, God is still good. He is cheering for us, just as a dad is cheering for his son who just tripped on the soccer field and missed the ball, "Keep going son. Don't give up!" Heart and action change lives.

We have a decision to make at every juncture, a choice as to how we will proceed. I found myself with a new phrase, "It's all good." Truthfully, this started out as an active way to convince myself and others around me that it was going to be okay, no matter how it turned out. It has since become my mantra, that I truly believe. It's all good, because we have a God who wants us to live life fulfilled and accepting of all that is. It's all God.

Life experience is a grand teacher. Once I saw God in action, fulfilling plans with results that were more magnificent than I could have dreamed up, it was easier to remember that God is good all the time. It is a comfort to know that God's got this too! Place it all in God's in-basket and *leave it there* for Him to complete.

II Corinthians 5:7
For we live by faith, not by sight.

What has God unexpectedly provided for you in the past?

_____

_____

_____

_____

_____

_____

_____

_____

_____

_____

_____

_____

_____

_____

_____

_____

... believe in you ...

We are all as different as the snowflakes, and how amazing is that! God created us each with unique talents and gifts that He intends for us to use as we praise and rejoice in Him and celebrate His gift of grace to us.

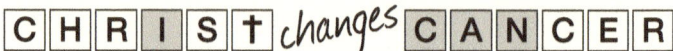

It is okay to be confident in your ability to overcome and to be your best! God has our back, which makes us super heroes with His special powers. Use this time of rebirth from a difficult time to explore your special strengths given to you by God. Be super today!

Actively look for ways to share yourself with others, as Jesus did. He walked with sinners. We are all sinners and continue to make mistakes, but we have a new outlook and a new lease on life because of God and Christ's sacrifice for our sins. Take time to reflect on our weaknesses and those challenges put before us. Ask God for wisdom and encouragement in those areas.

Find your center, your peace, your joy in knowing the final outcome is with God... whenever that time may come. Awesome joys and unimaginable peace await us on the other side. The happiness and opportunities we experience here on earth are only a tiny fraction of what is to come. Acknowledge the Creator and **commit** to His will.

Keep your eyes focused on God's promise of eternal life after this human existence. Think of a toddler running to retrieve a new, shiny toy. One who will not stop heading toward the goal, even if she falls down. God is the super power that moves our gears, the genius that creates our motivation and the wisdom that keeps our feet balanced on the ground. What will God's Holy Spirit guide me to do today that will bring me closer to Him and my brothers and sisters in Christ? Christ showed much compassion to others in need.

II Timothy 1:9

He has saved us and called us to a holy life—not because of anything we have done but because of his own purpose and grace.

What talents and gifts has God given to you?

_____

_____

_____

_____

_____

_____

_____

_____

_____

_____

_____

_____

_____

_____

_____

_____

⋯ *piece of life* ⋯

*As you progress through your treatment and recovery,
find a Bible verse or story, a song, a poem, a book or
other meaningful piece of life that will keep you going
in the darkest times. This journal may comfort you.*

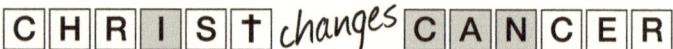

There are still incidents that trip me on my path. I am going strong, then stopped short with a negative thought or a painful experience. During these times, prayer, song and inspiration push me through the darkness to the warm sun on the other side.

It was welcoming, like an old friend. The song, "What Faith Can Do," by Kutless, lifted my spirits many, many times. Peace falls over me at the sound of the first few chords. When I am glum, the words inspire me and remind me how great God is. "Broken hearts become brand new, that's what faith can do." My heart has been broken and faith is the overcomer. God is speaking to me through their words.

The long-running TV show with Ty Pennington, "Extreme Home Makeover," reminded me that I am not the only one going through tough times. Cancer is just one of many tragic diseases and catastrophic events that severely affect lives of all ages. There is a common thread throughout. Each new home was a fresh start from a dismal situation from a health crisis or difficult life circumstance.

That new beginning would not be possible without the struggle. We are all survivors of something. We are survivors as long as there is air to breathe and a sun to rise. Love and live loved, regardless of your circumstances. Live well and **create** a new reality. Consider listening to a Christian radio station. Spend time with encouraging and God-affirming words set to music. Connect with "your" song. Our persona is, in part, defined by what we listen to on a daily basis.

Galations 5:22-23

But the fruit of the Spirit is love, joy, peace, forbearance, kindness, goodness, faithfulness, gentleness and self-control.

What meaningful piece of life deeply matters to you?

_____

_____

_____

_____

_____

_____

_____

_____

_____

_____

_____

_____

_____

_____

_____

_____

*Technology has progressed over the years and
medical advancements continue to arise.
Use these to your advantage, but take the time
to research what is best for you and your family.*

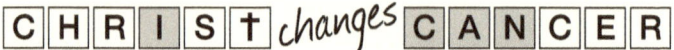

I thank God for my doctors, my treatment and my ongoing care. Pray for guidance and **continue** to research the plan that is best for you. He created our brains, the ability to discover, to invent and to treat illness. Pray for the best doctor and treatment for your cancer. Be assertive and ask questions. Research online. Pray with paper and pen to write questions down *before* your doctor visits. It is your responsibility for the body God gave to you.

My first surgeon consultation resulted in complete frustration, as he obviously had not yet read my chart and argued with me about the existence of nodules on both sides. My second opinion surgeon wanted to leave the right half of my thyroid, as only the left was showing questionable. In reality, it was the only half biopsied.

God is our **coach**. After hours of research, online chats and personal discussions with other thyroid cancer survivors, we decided to have a Total Thyroidectomy. I was going to be on meds for life anyway. We emphatically put this in writing. I remember Aaron stating "jokingly" to my surgeon as I drifted off to sleep, "No matter how good it looks, remove the entire thyroid, or I will hunt you down."

The follow-up biopsy revealed cancer on both sides and *not* in the nodules, even though the surgeon indicated the right half *looked* healthy. We thankfully avoided a second surgery. Whether you read it, heard it or it seems like common sense, *do not assume anything!* Seek counsel from multiple sources and decide what is best for you.

Proverbs 15:21-22

Folly brings joy to one who has no sense, but whoever has understanding keeps a straight course. Plans fail for lack of counsel, but with many advisers they succeed.

What research have you done regarding your cancer?

_____

_____

_____

_____

_____

_____

_____

_____

_____

_____

_____

_____

_____

_____

_____

_____

··· *sooner than later* ···

If your body is telling you something is not right, do not wait for it to go away. Seek a professional opinion or two. Early detection of cancer and lots of other diseases is key. Ask family and friends for referrals to trusted doctors.

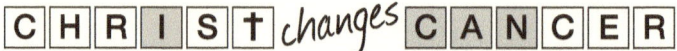

C H R I S t *changes* C A N C E R

I praise God for the early detection of my cancer. An appointment for bronchitis turned into cause for concern. My doctor was out, so I was seen by another. He felt a nodule in my neck. More tests were completed indicating cancer, and my journey had begun.

At a follow-up appointment with my regular doctor to get anxiety meds, he could not even feel the nodule. Scarey for me then, but comforting now. God knew the outcome and is fully **capable** of caring for me. I know, though, that my cancer would not have been detected early if I had not done my part by seeking professional care.

Resist your fear of the unknown and call today to schedule an appointment. It is better to know the cause and seek treatment than to allow it to destroy your body and weigh you down emotionally.

If you fear financial strain, research to find the best solution for you. Call your insurance, contact doctors at hospitals that offer financial aid, join a clinical trial or campaign for funds. Putting your head in the sand will only prolong the pain, and possibly, end your life early. Our medical finance journey has been frustrating and overwhelming at times. Take it one day at a time. Ask for hardship assistance and payment plans. Do not give up. Pray for God's will. He provides.

If you are not feeling well on a daily basis, how can you be living a full life for God? Check it out. Who knows? Maybe your ailment is minor, requiring a simple fix, and allowing you to get back to living a healthy, **complete**, joyous life, purposeful and rewarding.

I John 4:18

There is no fear in love. But perfect love drives out fear, because fear has to do with punishment. The one who fears is not made perfect in love.

What symptoms were you experiencing?

_____

_____

_____

_____

_____

_____

_____

_____

_____

_____

_____

_____

_____

_____

_____

_____

··· live through it ···

*Medical lingo, legal jargon, contractual jumbo...
just tell me in layman's term what that means.
Unless we are educated in a specific field, the
terminology is just plain difficult to understand.*

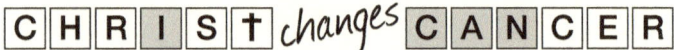

Papillary Thyroid Carcinoma (multi-foci, 0.7 x 0.5 cm, 0.6 x 0.4 cm, 0.4 x 0.4 cm) with tall cell features.

Tumors located in right and left lobes. Tumors confined to thyroid gland with no capsule or lymphovascular invasion.

Additional pathologic findings: Goiter, Hashimoto's Thyroiditis, Nodular Hyperplasia with Focal Hurthle Cell changes. According to the Mayo Clinic, Hurthle cell cancer is a rare form of thyroid cancer that can be more aggressive than other forms.

Did your eyes gloss over as you read this? Mine did too, but with tears and perplexity. This was the Surgical Pathology Report, but it reflected similar sentiments of the initial diagnosis.

Wow! The medical terms meant nothing. All I heard was cancer, rare, aggressive. Cry, cry and cry some more. It is okay to cry. Then, get on with it! Pray and research, talk and pray some more. Get real and find out what your diagnosis means. It is challenging and scarey, like facing a robber with a gun at your head.

Shoot for the moon. God is with you and wants peace for you at all times. Cancer is just one more thing in a list of many that you will face throughout your life. Enjoy and **celebrate** life every day we have! One day, there may be a cure for cancer. Until then and even when, God is our cure to a good life and His promises no matter what unfortunate and unhappy circumstances may arise.

John 14:27

Peace I leave with you; my peace I give you. I do not give to you as the world gives. Do not let your hearts be troubled and do not be afraid.

What is the technical name of your cancer or disease?

_____

_____

_____

_____

_____

_____

_____

_____

_____

_____

_____

_____

_____

_____

_____

··· all are survivors ···

Whether cancer, rape, suicide, marital strife, financial woes, domestic violence, addiction, illness, death, school and work drama, family tension... there is one solution... God. We are all survivors and worthy of a good life!

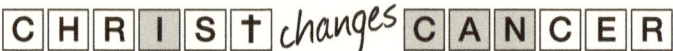

When enduring difficult, uphill battles, it is easy to question the win. But if you are reading this passage, you are victorious. You have survived another day. It is now time to claim that victory and live life to the fullest and be joyous in the life that is yours. Keep walking, keep climbing the hill. Rejoice in the small wins in the race of life.

So many times I have wasted my energy, debating God's will for me. Pray, seek counsel, make a plan, find peace and expect the plan to change. Repeat. Take a deep breath, ***chill***, and know God's got it. Survivors, of all sorts of life challenges, become comrades and life-long friends. There is a special bond. Look for others who have succeeded in the fight you are facing today. Ask for advice.

This life is tough. Watch the news for five minutes, and we see much sadness and hardship. The tragic events at the Twin Towers, the Boston Marathon and in Paris were horrific. However, victory and triumph over challenge is evident. Although we will never forget the loss, individuals and communities came together in support and healing of survivors, and remembrance of loved ones.

Pray for emotional peace and forgiveness during these difficult times. He will strengthen our resolve to overcome the grief and anger. Forgive those who hurt you. Each of us are responsible for our own decisions, some which will require us to acknowledge our mistakes. Avoid the temptation to let the actions of others define you. Seek to ***connect*** with the Almighty, let go of burdens and choose freedom.

Luke 6:37-38

Do not judge, and you will not be judged. Do not condemn, and you will not be condemned. Forgive, and you will be forgiven. Give and it will be given to you.

What other life circumstances make you a survivor?

_____

_____

_____

_____

_____

_____

_____

_____

_____

_____

_____

_____

_____

_____

_____

... the bad guy ...

I am still learning how to hear God. He gladly tells us what our next step should be, but we have to listen and then act, despite our fears and lack of complete understanding. Just like the hero and the villain, God and Satan both exist.

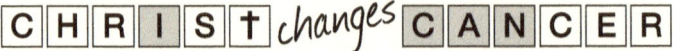

Ever have days when nothing goes right? Me too. A normal day can emotionally feel like running into a brick wall over and over. That could be Satan and his wily ways, enjoying laying snares in our path to throw us off our game. He is smart and on a mission to separate our minds from God. Satan will persist with subtle, seemingly innocent happenings. Sometimes we bring pain to our own lives and others by making poor choices. These are not of God, but He might stand back and let us handle it. Like a parent raising a teenager. The teen wants independence and opportunities for freedom of choice. Adolescence brings lessons that must be experienced and learned to become productive and responsible members of society. We must place God as #1 in our lives. All else revolves around Him and comes from Him.

Unfortunate, tragedy and hardship does not equal bad people or necessarily bad choices. The "devil on your shoulder" would like you to believe such nonsense. But my experience has taught me that bad things happen to great people every day! Bad circumstances and rebellious people happened to Jesus, but he never once sinned. What an amazing example of faith, love and forgiveness. Imagine Him on the **cross**... mocked, beaten and left to die by other human beings.

Satan wants to destroy us, but God remains in control. At His return, Satan's reign will end. Until then, Satan is sneaky like a mouse. Just when life is working out, there is a turn for the worse. Satan or coincidence? Could be either, but God will prevail in the end.

I Peter 5:8

Be alert and of sober mind. Your enemy the devil prowls around like a roaring lion looking for someone to devour.

What do you believe you are hearing from God?

_____

_____

_____

_____

_____

_____

_____

_____

_____

_____

_____

_____

_____

_____

_____

_____

··· words to paper ···

Being a believer and talking openly about your connection to and relationship with God does not make you a religious fanatic. It confirms your trust, belief and faith in a higher power. Be proud and share your love for Him.

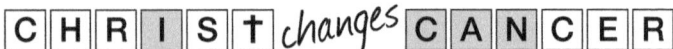

C H R I S † *changes* C A N C E R

Think of your best friend, maybe even your spouse. You trust them, right? You believe they will act in your best interest. That is what friends and parents try to do. God even more so. He is our biggest fan. Talk God up, like you would a friend who sent you flowers or wrote you an encouraging note. God is on our side and wants us to be happy, as we share the fulfillment of our dreams with Him.

He asks us to "armor up" daily, in order to take a stand against Satan. In the Bible, the book of Ephesians is a letter to the people of the Ephesian Church. It was written by a man named Paul who was one of the Apostles, New Testament men sent by God to preach the gospel of good news. Paul was a man of God, but he was not a perfect man. His story, like ours, was one of belief, faith and **choice**.

I believe we are here for a purpose, both men and women of Biblical times and now. Are our books all that different from those writings in the Bible? Being a graphic designer, I am a visual learner. I see the story acted out in my head, with people, places, smells and even emotions I might feel, like Christ sitting next to me in a time of need.

Paul wrote what God led him to write, to encourage and to share his experience. Are we so different? Words to paper. Thoughts to sentences, nouns and verbs, just like today. We have more advanced tech, but the process and the purpose is the same. God's armor gives us strength, but we have to take it up. He tells us to stand firm, with truth, righteousness, readiness, faith, salvation and the Word of God.

Ephesians 6:10-11

Finally, be strong in the Lord and in His mighty power. Put on the full armor of God, so that you can take your stand against the devil's schemes.

What words can you write of love and belief in God?

_____

_____

_____

_____

_____

_____

_____

_____

_____

_____

_____

_____

_____

_____

_____

··· over the falls ···

A sermon by Pastor Jeff Broadnax was epic for me. His gift of analogies and real life stories, brings God's purpose for us close to my heart and relates it intricately to this life. Sharing God's promise of grace to all is our purpose.

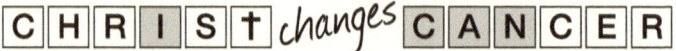

Terrified, I now send my anxiety "over the falls." God willing and God leading, His words in this book will leave the safety of my heart. My fears and my doubt will be faced. This is His will. When He leads you to your devine appointments, do you run and hide? It is time for me to wrap up my fear, doubt and shame and stuff them in a glass bottle for the water fall of life. May it crash to the bottom in tiny, little pieces and release my misguided restraint. Thanks for the words of wisdom and encouragement Pastor Jeff!

The thought of considering myself an author is intimidating to me, but not to God. He already knows who we are. He deliberately created each and every human and each for specific purpose. He knows our imperfections and our weaknesses. These bring us humility and understanding of others with the same. He knows our strengths and our talents. These bring us joy and acceptance in the celebration of others with the same. He made us, so He already knows. I am challenging my tendencies of perfectionism and procrastination.

Unabandoned freedom is what I pray for, but it scares me to the core. Why do I still question His will? It is because we are human. We are short-sighted, because what is to come is so incredible and beyond our human understanding. The song "I **Can** Only Imagine" by MercyMe highlights this point. God waits for us to feel His "nudges" and to share our imperfect and failure-filled lives with others. Give up control and open our minds to awe-inspiring possibilities, here on earth and much more beyond the grave.

Acts 20:24

However, I consider my life worth nothing to me; my only aim is to finish the race and complete the task the Lord Jesus has given me—the task of testifying to the good news of God's grace.

What leap of faith in your life is waiting on you?

_____

_____

_____

_____

_____

_____

_____

_____

_____

_____

_____

_____

_____

_____

_____

_____

... delay or purpose ...

*This book has been months in the making.
Words flowing at the oddest times, scribbled on whatever
scrap of paper I could find when God led me to do so. There
were more pages to write than I ever considered possible.*

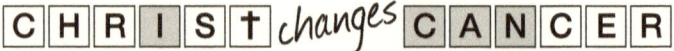

This passage is written one week after "over the falls." This book did not go to the publisher as soon as I had hoped. Typical delays again... ear and sinus infections, car troubles, work to complete, volunteer responsibilities to fulfill, finances to wrangle... and it was put off again. We struggle with procrastination of things that make us uncomfortable. This does. Who am I? I am far from a Biblical scholar, nor highly intelligent. I do not claim to know everything. In fact, I find myself full of questions and uncertainty.

Many times, there have been road blocks and pit falls, which initially felt like valid reasons to give up whatever mountain was being climbed that day. In hind sight, they turned out to be blessings in disguise. God does not expect us to be perfect, nor should we. He knows we will mess up, which is often how we learn.

Overcoming obstacles, heartache and pain often teaches us valuable lessons, strengthening our resolve to do better and to adjust our life trajectories. Our challenge is to listen for God, verifying if the delay is part of the journey requiring patience, or procrastination requiring motivation. Pastor Jeff shared with us in a sermon, not to leave a legacy, but to live a legacy, with God leading the way.

This earthly journey is not about me. It is all about God in me, and in you. He is waiting for us to give it all over to Him. With God in charge, what do I have to fear? God is **certain**. Keep listening for His guidance and His gifts. Let others see God in all that we do.

Philippians 1:6

Being confident of this, that He who began a good work in you will carry it on to completion until the day of Christ Jesus.

What excuses do you use as you hold back from big things?

_____

_____

_____

_____

_____

_____

_____

_____

_____

_____

_____

_____

_____

_____

_____

_____

_____

··· *live a legacy* ···

This reflection is about a man, Pastor John Halford, who lived his legacy. God called him home. We celebrated his life and the blessings God gave him... his family and all those who he touched in person, in writing and in spirit.

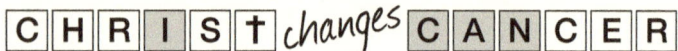

This book's cover photo was taken on the beautiful October day of John's funeral. It reminds me of God's presence, shining His light.

Six months prior to his death, John was diagnosed with stage four esophageal **cancer**. Thousands around the world prayed to God for his healing. Word of his cancer was the catalyst to the writing of these pages. A simple thought, "What can I say to offer hope, peace and loving support to his daughters, Becki and Judy and their families, having dealt with cancer myself?" My heart tugged, ripped by many emotions. That day at church was the beginning of these words to paper and a new journey that I never dreamed possible.

John lived his legacy, within a God-inspired life, challenging the traditional and the expected, with a fresh look through God's eyes. As a Pastor, he traveled and spoke where God led him, encouraging the weak and confused. He listened and asked questions, inspiring faith-filled conversations. I read an article written by him in our church magazine, while in my early 20s. It was a time of hypocrisy and confusion, with our church transitioning, uncertainty in my beliefs, relationship questions and other pastors' disregard for me.

If not for Pastor John Halford and our local Pastor John Karlson leading Aaron and I to Jesus and His grace, we would not be attending church today. We thank God for both of these witty, genuine men of God, who confirmed in teaching us that Christ died on the cross for our sins, and God's gift of grace frees us from them.

John 3:16

For God so loved the world that He gave His one and only Son, that whoever believes in Him shall not perish but have eternal life.

What legacy are you leaving in the hearts of others?

_____

_____

_____

_____

_____

_____

_____

_____

_____

_____

_____

_____

_____

_____

_____

_____

_____

_____

... forged by people ...

*Pay it forward. Be the change. Make an impactful
difference to those who God places in your world.
My spiritual essence, confidence and journey has been
forged by people from God. People make a difference.*

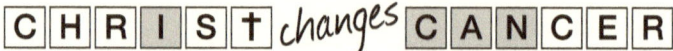

Even those events I would rather forget were positively spun, or intentionally worked out for good by God. We felt God's spirit and grace working from His love in action through family and friends.

It is simple. Love God. Love others. God does not want, nor need us to earn our place. He has already given it. Acknowledge and praise Him, for all He has given. Living a life of love and outreach is our pleasure and our thanks for so many blessings. Find your passions and live them daily. Jeremy Camp's song, "Same Power," reminds me that I am not alone, but my Father's power is in me.

My faith has grown exponentially as I grow older and experience life, good and bad. Our family and friends have been key! Our church family is one we would not trade for anything. Sunday is a day to rejuvenate with messages and connections with our brothers and sisters in **Christ**. It is a time to unite with God in outreach to others.

Feeling lonely or looking for spiritual support? Find a church to call home, not for the place, but for the people. If you have been hurt in the past, forgive, and ask God to help you find another church home.

A church is like a hospital for healing, not a courtroom. Having been judged, this sentiment settles well in my heart. Let us seek spiritual help and healing from God and His people, so our lives are His all week long. Let us offer spiritual help and healing through God to His people. Reach out to others, and offer a welcoming, encouraging, accountable testimony to all of God's children. God forgives all!

Hebrews 10:25

Not giving up meeting together, as some are in the habit of doing, but encouraging one another—and all the more as you see the Day approaching.

What help can you offer to a fellow son or daughter of God?

_____

_____

_____

_____

_____

_____

_____

_____

_____

_____

_____

_____

_____

_____

_____

_____

The more I consider my path, the more evident it is that God is present. He wants to be near to our hearts, a conscious presence every second of every day, a go-to in joy and praise, as well as in pain and uncertainty.

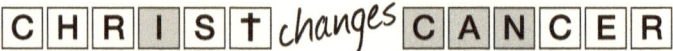

When the first words of this book flowed from my brain, almost unwillingly, I also did a random "Google" search for a publishing company. This task had proved most difficult with my first book attempt, which is 98% complete, still sitting on my computer. Our youngest, Noelle, was one year old when we completed the photos of that simple, photographic counting book. She is now nine. It is past time for me to be **confident** in God's plan for me.

After connecting with Westbow Press, my representative, Maurice, explained the process and inquired about my venture. I was timid, of course, and it has taken more time than planned to get to this point. Maurice continued to call me as requested, encouraging me and keeping me motivated with this book venture. God was evident in the weekly brief phone calls of a man I hope one day to meet. He encouraged me by simple words and continues to be my **champion**. In the course of our conversations, I shared my story of cancer, and he has shared his life experiences of his mom's and sister's cancers. Early on, I asked him to pray for our friend who just passed away. Maurice specifically told me he would head to the prayer closet as soon as we finished talking, which filled my heart with God's love.

Despite life happenings, regular excuses, and "call me next week" replies on my part, Maurice was a blessing placed by God. Even with the support of our family and friends, God knew I needed the gentle, weekly prodding of an objective, encouraging friend to hold me accountable and keep me moving toward completion of this book.

Philippians 2:2

Then make my joy complete by being like-minded, having the same love, being one in spirit and of one mind.

What do you lack confidence in pursuing?

_____
_____
_____
_____
_____
_____
_____
_____
_____
_____
_____
_____
_____
_____
_____
_____
_____

gift of words

I believe God puts people in the same room for destined, amazing reasons. The ladies gathered around the table one evening, from ages 20s to 40s. Each had so much to give. I saw God through them and felt Him in the room.

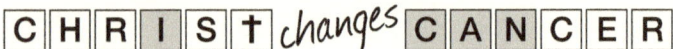

C H R I S t *changes* C A N C E R

I graduated Summa Cum Laude, and yet reading was a chore for me. Years back I joined a book **club**, purely for social reasons. A group of friends, brought together by a talented woman named Lee Lander, encouraged me, contributed to my well-being, brought the books alive and sparked my interest for reading the stories of others. We first read "Hind's Feet" by Hannah Hurnard. My take-away was a renewed connection with God and my spiritual growth. Forgiveness and faith change lives if we are open to God's Word. Written words **contribute** to growth by offering new perspectives.

I am thankful for those inspired by God to write what He leads them to share in journal, in book testimony or in the form of a motivational movie. Consider God in writings of all kinds, keeping the Bible as our firm foundation. It all comes back to Him and His Word. Jesus is the way and the truth and the life. God gives us many ways to find Him.

The "Shack" by William Paul Young was the next book that truly made me think about my specific place in this life and what I truly believed. To my dear friend, Fian Kunesh, please keep putting books in front of me. She is an amazing reader and teacher. God is so good to have joined us in mission with our church youth. Her extensive reading has brought us many valuable words of wisdom in the form of books.

Pick up a book, read alone or with friends. Maybe write your own. God speaks to us directly via the Bible, just as He does through His sons and daughters here on earth with His gift of words. Read on!

John 14:6

Jesus answered, "I am the way and the truth and the life. No one comes to the Father except through me. If you really know me, you will know my Father as well."

What books have made a difference in your life?

_____

_____

_____

_____

_____

_____

_____

_____

_____

_____

_____

_____

_____

_____

_____

_____

··· *anger steals joy* ···

Who are you angry at today? Family or friend, the guy that cut you off in traffic, the sales rep that made no sense? That person is also a child of God. Be respectful, calm and kind. Be responsible, and yet forgiving, just like Jesus.

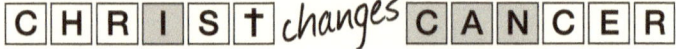

Coming home from a challenging day, the kids had not yet completed homework or chores. Frustration high from the exhaustion of the day, it was easy to get angry, causing my heart to race, my head to hurt and to physically feel ill. I allowed the stress of my day to influence my response to their actions. It was not good for any of us. Hard to admit, but this life gets the best of me at times. Our kids are amazing, but they also face stress and obstacles of their own.

God has given us the blessed privilege of teaching our children and setting a good example. Acknowledge when we fall short, apologize and do better next time. Listen first; stay calm; engage realistic, age-appropriate expectations and predetermined consequences; and speak the love of Christ. Rejoice in the help of grandparents, aunts, uncles, and the whole village, when you need a break. Consider times we messed up and hoped others would be merciful.

Anger steals joy. My evening played to a negative tune. What if I had handled it with more finesse? Choose our paths and walk as Jesus would have. Wow! That is tough, and we will not always do it right. God is working with me on this one, as I am a work-in-progress.

What do my words and my actions say about God? Is it the same message Jesus sent? The movie, "Do You Believe?" poses a valid question. One asks, "If you were ever accused of being a Christian, would there be enough evidence to convict you?" Seek honor and be a ***class*** player in the game of life. Forgive and live forgiven.

James 1:19-20

My dear brothers and sisters, take note of this: Everyone should be quick to listen, slow to speak and slow to become angry, because human anger does not produce the righteousness that God desires.

What makes you angry that you could handle better?

_____

_____

_____

_____

_____

_____

_____

_____

_____

_____

_____

_____

_____

_____

_____

It helps me to connect physical items with spiritual concepts, especially when sharing God's word with youth. Is God real? Some say no, as science says God is not visible. I say yes, because His Spirit is in my heart and soul.

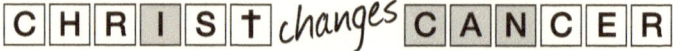

C H R I S t *changes* C A N C E R

There are many life experiences that convict me God is real. There is just no other explanation. The truths of these events defy any other reasoning for me. The song "We Believe" by the Newsboys asks us all, "Do you believe in God the Father, Jesus Christ, the Holy Spirit, the Crucifixion and the Resurrection?" Does the wind exist if we cannot see it? I believe the wind exists, as I see the leaves on the trees and the waves in the ocean move. I believe God exists, as I have seen His Spirit "move" in my life many times.

In one teen lesson at church, each received a red bell, symbolizing the blood of Christ, with a blue "Believe" ribbon. As they ring it, I hope their hearing the expected sound every time will remind them that their life experiences and faith in God's spiritual existence is *just as certain.* He wants a deep, personal relationship with every one of us. We must affirm our beliefs and define it personally with a Biblical foundation! God is **constant**, so must be our beliefs, irregardless of cultural trends or others' convictions. God is our only compass!

Christ died in his 30s. What an impact His life had for us within His short human life. Remember John 1. God is here and has always been here. Christ lived a perfect human life, but there was pain and suffering (Matthew 27). Life brings emotional and spiritual growth, just as an adult is more mature than a child. We look forward to the day when there is no more suffering... when Jesus Christ returns, and we begin a new spiritual life with Him forever. What do you believe?

Romans 15:13

May the God of hope fill you with all joy and peace as you trust in Him, so that you may overflow with hope by the power of the Holy Spirit.

What do you believe about God, Jesus and the Holy Spirit?

_____

_____

_____

_____

_____

_____

_____

_____

_____

_____

_____

_____

_____

_____

_____

_____

_____

··· *who is worthy* ···

We are all worthy of a great life, but not by anything we have done. God's grace covers all our sin to live a life of freedom in Him. View our lives through God's giant, hopeful magnifying glass and not just a tiny, hopeless, pinhole lens.

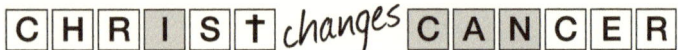

C H R I S t *changes* C A N C E R

Coming home from John's funeral, Nicole shared a part of her amazing story. She will turn 18 this November and begin her adult life. What a blessing God has given us in her. She is relying on God to lead her journey. It is not always easy, even though she makes it seem so. Case in point, she was frustrated by some friends who had commented, "You have such a perfect life." or "What do you have to worry about?" *Everyone* has garbage to deal with. We all need to manage it as best we can. Our attitudes and reliance on God matter.

God is working in her. She gets up and wears her beautiful smile inside and out, despite the emotional realities of my cancer, her own precancerous moles, limited finances including foreclosure struggles due to medical bills, academics, relationships, unfair life lessons, and challenges in sports including politics and injuries. Through it all, she has found her voice and her confidence to walk through it with God by her side. Every person on this planet has "tough stuff."

God reminded me of a reality that afternoon through Nicole. The grass is not greener on the other side, even though her peers thought so. Do not wish our own lives away, to frivolously wish upon another's life. Find peace at this very moment, where you are, who you are, what you own, what you owe, who loves you, what blessings abound, most importantly, what you **cherish**. Be thankful and joyous in the life you have right now, with all the good and the bad! Tomorrow is a new day. Get up and make better what you can.

II Corinthians 9:8

And God is able to bless you abundantly, so that in all things at all times, having all that you need, you will abound in every good work.

What do you treasure the most in this life?

_____

_____

_____

_____

_____

_____

_____

_____

_____

_____

_____

_____

_____

_____

_____

⋯ *friends are forever* ⋯

When pregnant for the first time and incredibly nervous about the concept of a baby (9 lb. 7 oz.) exiting my body, I remember thinking, "If millions of woman can deliver a baby, so can I." It got me through.

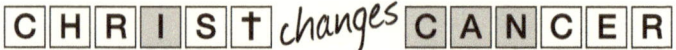

The same holds true for anything. If millions of people can survive cancer, so can I. If millions of people can write a book, so can I. Preface this with the knowledge of God's will (not mine), and He will guide you through any challenge. I used this as incentive to dig deep and to keep trying, no matter what came.

My husband, Aaron, and I welcomed the incredible support of family and friends. Aaron shared his biggest sorrow was being unable to take away my discomfort. Remember... sometimes it is the simple hug and the holding of a hand that gets us through a difficult spell. Other times it is the persistent, attentive questions being asked of the doctor and gentle reminders to the nurses, that help us know we are in good hands while we are incapable of caring for ourselves. It is knowing our kids are cared for while we cannot do so, that brings peace. Lying in bed is tough for a type A soul like me.

To the caregivers who accept the burden of diving deep into the trenches with a loved one with cancer, *thank you!* In our fear, our pain and our focus on ourselves, we often forget to say these two meaningful words. You have *chosen* to be there for us, with stressful and lonely nights, wondering how it will all end. God knows *your* pain too. To family and friends of those facing cancer, *thank you* for your meaningful, heartfelt prayers; your time, gifts, cards, and homemade goodies; your **compassion**; and your sharing of God's love with those in need! You are appreciated and an answered prayer!

Luke 11:9

So I say to you: Ask and it will be given to you; seek and you will find; knock and the door will be opened to you.

What motivational, inspirational thoughts can you share?

_____

_____

_____

_____

_____

_____

_____

_____

_____

_____

_____

_____

_____

_____

... boost in confidence ...

From the day of my diagnosis, I have pondered the question, "Why do some die from cancer and others do not?" Lots of us have entertained this thought, but do not let it consume you. "Survivor's guilt" has no place in our hearts.

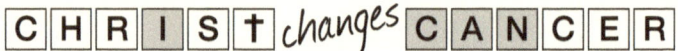

C H R I S t *changes* C A N C E R

Every day we must live for God and those we love, including those who have died. Human minds micromanage and narrow possibilities with a small, tunneled vision. God is so much bigger than this! He knows the big picture and all the joy to come! He shares our pain, suffering and sadness when we lose someone or feel like all is lost. We cannot be fearful and focus on length of this physical life. God plans a life with us for eternity and promises we will see them again.

When tragedies happen, we hear many stories of the kind, generous, perseverant, accepting, courageous, resilient and supportive spirit of mankind that lives on through the challenge. God is merciful and loving and does not see physical death in this life as an end. It is a magnificent beginning to the spiritual joy in the presence of our Almighty God. How fantastic! According to the Population Reference Bureau (prb.org), 56,759,000 people died worldwide just in 2014." It is the cycle of life and is guaranteed to happen to every person.

Do not let this get you down. *Celebrate your life and the lives of those who have passed.* God's grace allows us to live free from fear. Find **comfort** in the knowledge that we are not alone. Two quotes come to mind. "Leave this world a little better than you found it," by Robert Baden-Powell, founder of Scouting. And Helen Keller shared, "Alone we can do so little, together we can do so much?" I thank God for the knowledge of Him and His constant presence. Without His hope, this life would be a different, dismal journey for me.

Psalm 28:7

The Lord is my strength and my shield; my heart trusts in Him, and He helps me. My heart leaps for joy, and with my song I praise Him.

What joyful memories can you share of a life lived well?

_____

_____

_____

_____

_____

_____

_____

_____

_____

_____

_____

_____

_____

_____

_____

_____

_____

Today is the day. Do not let one more day pass without beginning your next challenge. Start small, with just one piece of the puzzle. One day at a time and one piece in place every day. Before you know it, you will complete your goal.

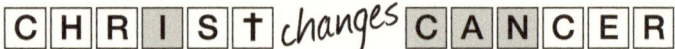

C H R I S T *changes* C A N C E R

It seems that until I make a clear stance in my head, choices are vague and elusive. Above all else, is God. He's got this! This very minute, give your heart, your soul and your body to Him. Thank Him, praise Him and serve Him as a cancer survivor. Join with your brothers and sisters in Christ, your brothers and sisters in survival of all the hardships we face. Affirm your commitment to Him and face each day with Him by your side, walking with you through the pain, the heartbreak and the victories, even small ones, won day by day.

Today could be my last day on earth. I will get up today, thankful for the opportunity, and live as God would have me do. Check out the song, "Try" by Colbie Caillat. "You don't have to try so hard... you don't have to bend until you break... you just have to get up." Be your God-created self and find your confidence in Him.

God not only likes you, He loves you and **cares** for you with all His heart. That is big! I believe with all my heart that God is real. He has a plan. It is time for us to rise to the challenge and live with our hearts wide open, with complete surrender! God's got this too!

It is our choice to participate in whatever comes our way. Dig deep and pull out whatever ounce of strength remains. If you find yourself sobbing in a fetal position, that's okay. **Cry** it out, then make a plan. Open your heart to Him. Then let Him take the lead. Celebrate the good, and deal with the bad and the ugly with a can-do, positive, accepting, fearless attitude.

Ephesians 2:10

For we are God's handiwork, created in Christ Jesus to do good works, which God prepared in advance for us to do.

What is God leading you to do this very day?

_____

_____

_____

_____

_____

_____

_____

_____

_____

_____

_____

_____

_____

_____

_____

_____

... change in perspective ...

We have talked at length about the ugly "c" word, cancer.
Now let us discuss the other 39 "c" words noted here.
It is time to change our perspective, to rethink our
strategy for life and living. Christ changes cancer!

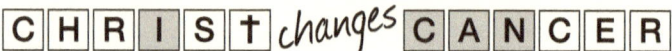

Take a look at my list of 40 positive, encouraging "c" words. There are others, but I found a connection with these words, which are found throughout the book in bold italic text.

Calling, calm, can, cancer, capable, cares, carry, celebrate, certain, champion, change, cheerful, cherish, chill, choice, Christ, church, clarity, class, club, coach, comfort, commit, compassion, complete, confident, confirm, connect, **conquer**, constant, content, continue, contribute, cope, courage, create, cross, cry, cuddle and cure.

Christ does change cancer. Take the journey with God, and He will guide you. Twist your brain around the possibility that cancer, or any other hardship, might just be a good thing. I believe cancer changed my life for the better. It can for you too.

Our journeys may be similar only in small ways, and our paths may only cross a few similar obstacles. My cancer experience may be remarkably unlike yours. However, the basics are the same. Love God, love others. Remember the fruit of God's Holy Spirit. Praise Him and be thankful. Forgive. Live loved, peaceful, content and faith-filled lives. Our journeys are the same in God's love.

Embrace all 40 "c" words in this book as positive, encouraging and inspirational. Act on them and engage their true meaning. Strive to embody all of these words, not just cancer. But embrace it too. The cancer and the daily victories are part of who you are. Turn CANCER into *CANCER*. Carry the cross and live as Jesus did here on earth.

Matthew 19:26

Jesus looked at them and said, "With man this is impossible, but with God all things are possible."

What do see differently now about the "cancer" word?

_____

_____

_____

_____

_____

_____

_____

_____

_____

_____

_____

_____

_____

_____

_____

_____

_____

··· crossword puzzle fun ···

There are 40 special "c" words to place within the crossword puzzle. You can find the word that belongs on the page noted below. It will be a word in bold italic.

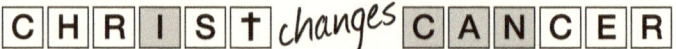

ACROSS		DOWN	
1	page 42	1	page 40
2	page 46	2	page 44
3	page 30	3	page 16
4	page 4	4	page 58
5	page 2	5	page 28
6	page 22	6	page 58
7	page 26	7	page 6
8	page 30	8	page 60
9	page 4	9	page 14
10	page 24	10	page 32
11	page 34	11	page 36
12	page 38	12	page 26
13	page 14	13	page 56
14	page 54	14	page 8
15	page 8	15	page 52
16	page 50	16	page 10
17	page 16	17	page 46
18	page 48	18	page 24
19	page 20	19	page 12
20	page 44	20	page 18

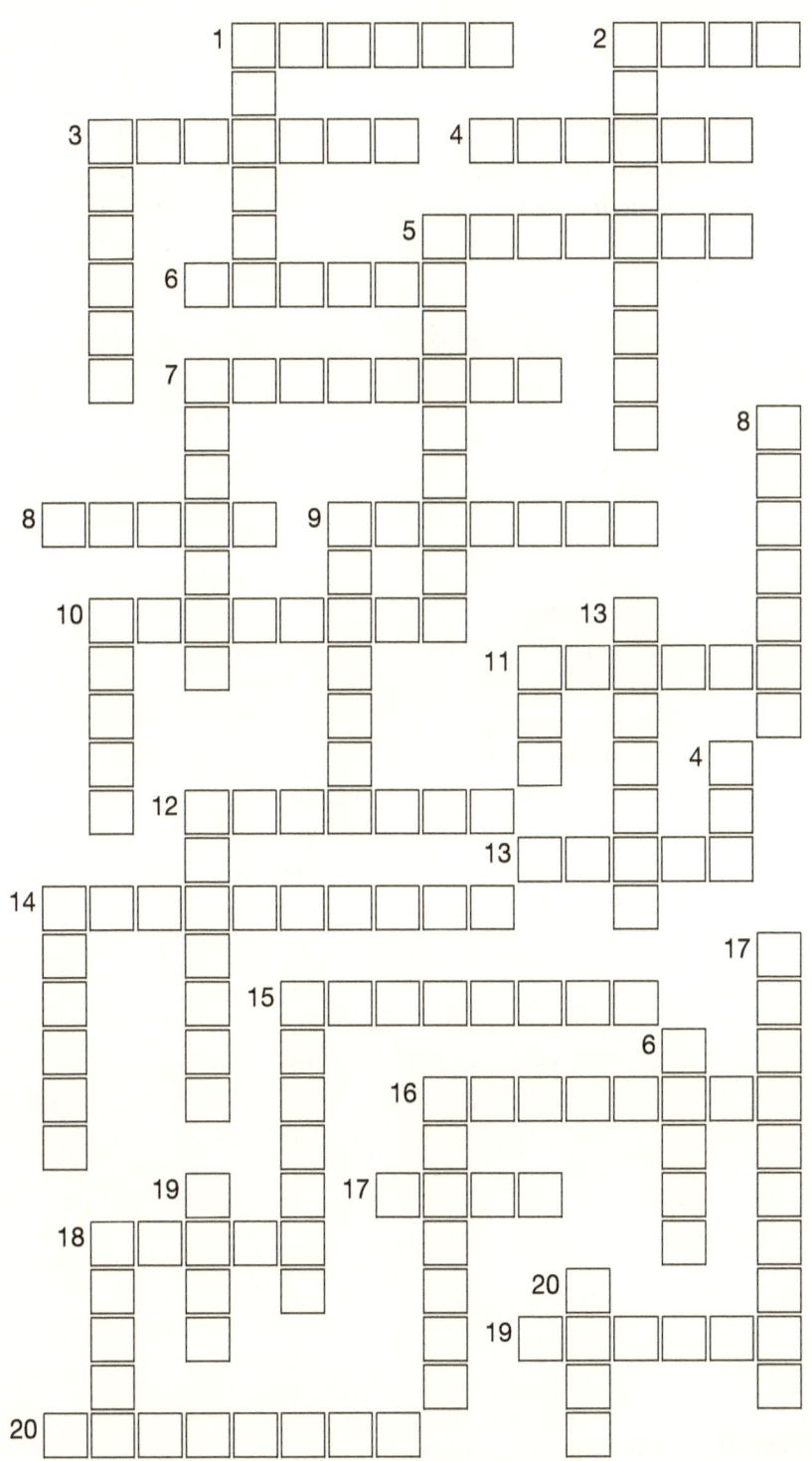

... word find challenge ...

There are 40 special "c" words to find amongst the letters in the word find. They are listed below in alphabetical order. Circle the word when you find it.

C H R I S T changes C A N C E R

calling	coach
calm	comfort
can	commit
cancer	compassion
capable	complete
cares	confident
carry	confirm
celebrate	connect
certain	conquer
champion	constant
change	content
cheerful	continue
cherish	contribute
chill	cope
choice	courage
Christ	create
church	cross
clarity	cry
class	cuddle
club	cure

```
E U N I T N O C B X G J S U Y I
Q A P O N R Z E D U O V M Q W O
K F E R A Z A P B C A P A B L E
M C O N T R I B U T E Y N T W C
I S C X S C B G D K P H E I U R
G E P R N A N Y C O N F I R M K
H C U E O I W O F N P U E A V R
R I E A C S B N I R E Q S T E Z
C H I L L C S Y B P L F B C D S
A X C M E O K A O D M V N T T K
L I F H X B B C W J G A O B N B
L V C H E A R E M Z C I H A E U
I A W B J E O A T Q K C M C D L
N T I R C B R N T A S H L O I C
G C U I T C F F D E E V W M F X
C R O P N O S L U R C R Y P N M
S H M N R N B X J L N O C A O T
C K F Q N T G A E Z V H P S C Z
O R I C H E R I S H E C M S N R
U V S C X N C O K C L A R I T Y
R B U E P T A T C P K O N O Y S
A C A R E S X O S A G C J N N O
G V D T B G W Z E R L V I A S P
E M V A C H U R C H A M Z W T I
L Q Y I U R K R D C N E P S R V
C H A N G E E S E G A H I J O S
O V U Z R U M L A S K R G L F S
M K P B Q D D O I V H N R U M A
M J S N X D J A F C R D H Y O L
I Y O P U Q I V W M U O K B C C
T C K C Z E T E L P M O C M R I
```

⋯ I am mighty ⋯

This just "might" be the title to my next book.
Our family was blessed to take a vacation last summer
to Virginia Beach. The ocean is amazing and the waves
spoke volumes to me again of the awesomeness of God.

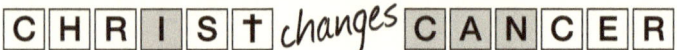

We are *all* mighty in unique ways. Without God, we are limited to our own physical strength. With God's Spirit, Power and Vision, *nothing* is impossible. In fact, with absolute freedom in His will, amazing and unbelievable accomplishments are possible and should be expected!

Close your eyes and envision a beautiful, sunny day at the beach, with powerful waves beating against the sandy shores. Even now, I can feel God's Spirit soar within, encourage and energize me, as I reminisce of the soothing and relaxing atmosphere. What a blessing!

The white sea gulls fly low overhead, carefree and shouting "be free" in their flight. The blue sky falling into the horizon reminds me that God's power is limitless, and so too can mine be. Sunset and sunrise, even through the mist, magnificently envelope me in the comfort that evening brings rest and morning brings a new day.

Joy and thankfulness rang true as our family enjoyed the beauty of God's creation and His presence in our lives. I visualize the single set of "Footprints in the Sand," as those of Christ carrying me (never leaving me), as the poem by Mary Stevenson brings to life.

As you walk with God, use the journal pages to express your feelings. I find writing is therapeutic. Do not let one thought fade away. If God leads you to write it, do so, even if it never leaves your house. If you are so inclined, send an email to share your short story of how God empowered you to be mighty. He may be leading my next book to include your short story in a series of testimonials in His name.

almightystory@gmail.com

I look forward to reading your story of faith and fulfillment
through belief in God, His Word and His presence in your life.
God is good, all the time. He is with you, as you read these words!

How has the Almighty empowered you to be mighty?

_____

_____

_____

_____

_____

_____

_____

_____

_____

_____

_____

_____

_____

_____

_____

··· *my story matters* ···

This is your space to write whatever you are feeling...
vent, share, praise, rhyme, wonder, explain, convict,
document, question. Put it here, then let God do the rest!

C H R I S t *changes* C A N C E R

_____

_____

_____

_____

_____

_____

_____

_____

_____

_____

_____

_____

Journal here. Write it down. Let it go.

_____

_____

_____

_____

_____

_____

_____

_____

_____

_____

_____

_____

_____

_____

_____

_____

_____

··· *tell me why* ···

*Jot down why you feel God is working in your life.
What changes are Christ helping you embrace through
your unique and specific cancer experiences?*

C H R I S † *changes* C A N C E R

_____

_____

_____

_____

_____

_____

_____

_____

_____

_____

_____

_____

Words to paper. New perspectives. I can do this.

_____

_____

_____

_____

_____

_____

_____

_____

_____

_____

_____

_____

_____

_____

_____

_____

_____

_____

_____

_____

_____

_____

_____

_____

_____

_____

_____

_____

_____

_____

_____

_____

_____

_____

_____

_____

_____

··· *peace and hope* ···

Write about what gives you peace in the moment and hope for the future. Share your convictions, give your testimony and honor those who have filled your heart through it all.

C H R I S t *changes* C A N C E R

_____

_____

_____

_____

_____

_____

_____

_____

_____

_____

_____

_____

Thankful things. A positive spirit. Reasons to believe.

_____

_____

_____

_____

_____

_____

_____

_____

_____

_____

_____

_____

_____

_____

_____

_____

_____

··· *God conquers all* ···

*All we accomplish, own and create belongs to Him. Our lives have definite purpose. Look through His mighty lens and put into words what **His** vision might look like for you.*

C H R I S t *changes* C A N C E R

_____

_____

_____

_____

_____

_____

_____

_____

_____

_____

_____

_____

Our lives are His. We are worthy in Him. Dream big.

_____

_____

_____

_____

_____

_____

_____

_____

_____

_____

_____

_____

_____

_____

_____

_____

_____

_____

_____

··· *motivation and action* ···

What motivates you? Who, why or what gives you a reason to jump out of bed in the morning? Enthusiasm for the finish line keeps us trudging up the hill, with God in front.

C H R I S t *changes* C A N C E R

_____

_____

_____

_____

_____

_____

_____

_____

_____

_____

_____

_____

Inspiration brings change. Be meaningful. Find joy.

_____

_____

_____

_____

_____

_____

_____

_____

_____

_____

_____

_____

_____

_____

_____

··· *face your fear* ···

Healthy fear keeps us safe. However, certain fears simply hold us back from God's will for us. Ask God, right now, to convict you of your purpose. What is He saying to you?

C H R I S t *changes* C A N C E R

_____

_____

_____

_____

_____

_____

_____

_____

_____

_____

_____

_____

Open your heart. Listen for Him. Let Him.

_____

_____

_____

_____

_____

_____

_____

_____

_____

_____

_____

_____

_____

_____

_____

_____

··· *power of one* ···

Track your goals. One year from today, you will be closer to, further from or still pondering the same intention. Goals are met one step, one word, one dollar, one pound at a time.

C H R I S T *changes* C A N C E R

_____

_____

_____

_____

_____

_____

_____

_____

_____

_____

_____

Be specific. Never give up. Accomplish much.

_____

_____

_____

_____

_____

_____

_____

_____

_____

_____

_____

_____

_____

_____

_____

_____

_____

_____

www.ingramcontent.com/pod-product-compliance
Lightning Source LLC
Chambersburg PA
CBHW050401290526
45786CB00003B/1082